DANGEROUS DRUGS

ALCOHOL

JEFF BURLINGAME

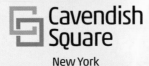

Cavendish
Square

New York

Published in 2014 by Cavendish Square Publishing, LLC
303 Park Avenue South, Suite 1247, New York, NY 10010

LIBRARY OF CONGRESS CATALOGING-IN-PUBLICATION DATA
Burlingame, Jeff.
Alcohol / Jeff Burlingame.
p. cm. — (Dangerous drugs)
Includes bibliographical references and index.
Summary: "Provides comprehensive information on the dangers of alcohol use"—Provided by publisher.
ISBN 978-1-60870-822-2 (hardcover)   ISBN 978-1-62712-058-6 (paperback)
ISBN 978-1-60870-828-4 (ebook)
1. Alcoholism—Juvenile literature. 2. Alcohol—Physiological effect—Juvenile literature.
I. Title. II. Series.
RC565.B88 2013
616.86´1—dc23
2011019152

EDITOR: Christine Florie   ART DIRECTOR: Anahid Hamparian   SERIES DESIGNER: Kristen Branch

EXPERT READER: John Schulenberg, PhD, Professor, Department of Psychology; Research Professor, Institute for Social Research, University of Michigan, Ann Arbor

Photo research by Marybeth Kavanagh

Cover photo by Sacramento Bee/MCT/Landov
The photographs in this book are used by permission and through the courtesy of: *SuperStock*: Photocuisine, 4; Cusp, 11; Kablonk, 41; *The Image Works*: Peter Hvizdak, 7; Andrew Lichtenstein, 8, 44; Bob Daemmrich, 12; Jeff Greenberg, 39; Rachel Epstein, 46; Syracuse Newspapers/Mike Greenlar, 55; *Corbis*: Photocuisine, 10; *Newscom*: Hulteng/MCT, 15; Ralph Notaro/Splash News, 50; *Phototake*: ISM, 18; *Getty Images*: Denis Boissavy/Taxi, 20; Joe Raedle, 26; Al Seib-Pool, 30; *Alamy*: Jeffrey Blackler, 22; Jeffrey Campbell, 35; *AP Images*: Frank Micelotta/PictureGroup, 32; *PhotoEdit Inc.*: Mary Kate Denny, 57. Most subjects in these photos are models.

Printed in the United States of America

CONTENTS

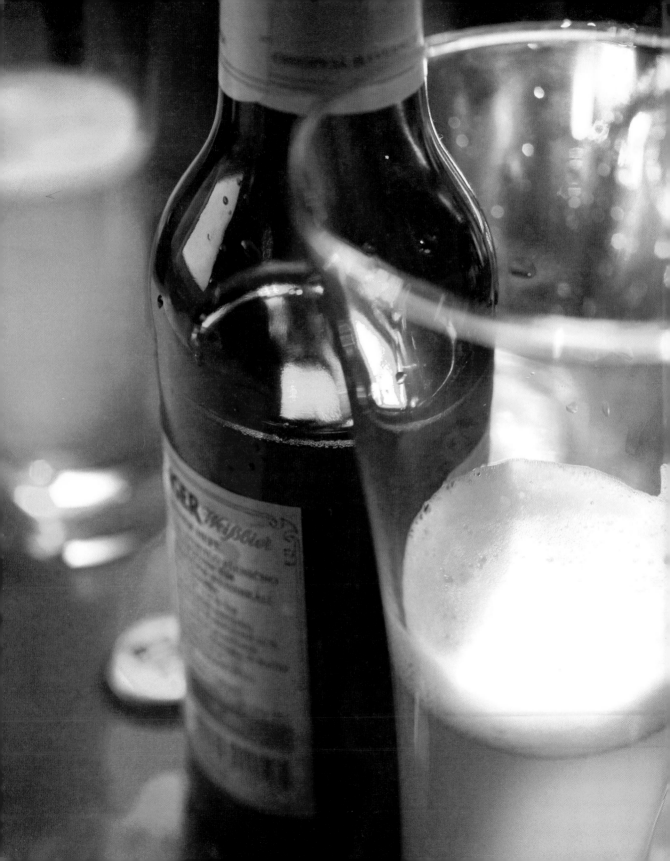

CHAPTER ONE

Illegal and Dangerous

ALCOHOL IS A POISONOUS DRUG. DRINKING it can damage a person's brain, liver, and heart. It can cause cancer of the colon, mouth, and throat; immune system disorders; and psychological issues such as anxiety and depression. It can even lead to suicide. More immediate effects can include blackouts, dizziness, and vomiting. If too much is consumed in one sitting, **alcohol poisoning** and death can occur. Each year, some 80,000 people die from causes related to excessive alcohol use. Alcohol can, and often does, shave years off a person's life. Still, most people drink it.

Left: Although one of the most dangerous drugs, alcohol is the most consumed drug in the United States.

Alcohol's effect on teen users often is even worse than it is on adults. Study after study has shown that drinking leads teens to engage in dangerous and risky behaviors. Teens who drink are more likely to have unprotected sex, which can lead to unwanted pregnancies or sexually transmitted diseases, which can be fatal. Teens who drink are more likely to be overweight than those who do not drink. Half of the drownings among male teens are due to alcohol use. Drinking also increases the chances that a teen will be involved in a homicide, suicide, or car accident. To top it off, alcohol is illegal for anyone under the age of twenty-one. Getting caught with it can lead to fines, arrests, suspension of driver's licenses, and criminal records. Drinking at a young age can also lead to alcohol dependence later in life. Teens who start drinking before age fifteen are four times more likely to develop an alcohol addiction than those who wait until they are twenty-one to have their first drink.

Still, many teens drink alcohol. According to the 2010 report "Monitoring the Future: National Survey on Drug Use" conducted by the University of Michigan, Ann Arbor, nearly four out of ten eighth graders have reported using alcohol at least once in their lifetimes. Almost half

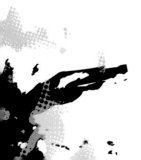

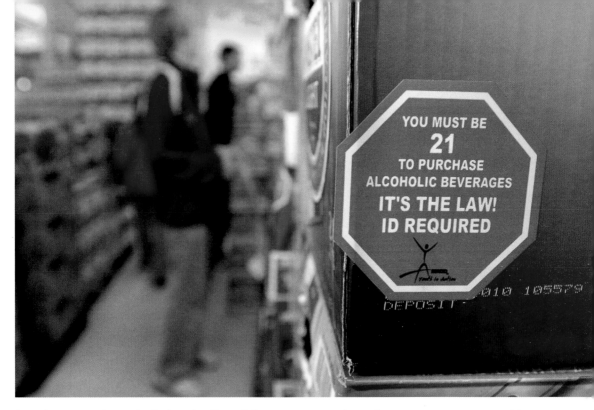

In order to purchase alcohol in the United States, you must be at least twenty-one years old.

of those—17 percent of all eighth graders—have reported being drunk at least once.

Today, more than half of adults age twenty-one or older drink alcohol at least once a month, and 20 percent of Americans drink excessively. Excessive drinking is defined as either having more than an average of two drinks a day for a man and one drink a day for a woman, or drinking more than five drinks on one occasion for a man or four drinks on one occasion for a woman.

Alcohol is the most widely used drug in the United States. It also is the drug of choice for America's adolescents, even though it is illegal for them to have it or drink it. An estimated 28 percent—nearly three out of ten, or 10.8 million people—of those ages twelve to twenty say they currently drink alcohol, and the number of reported users increases with age. Almost three out of four twelfth graders have tried alcohol, more than two out of five are current drinkers, and nearly six out of ten have reported being drunk at least once in their lives. A 2009 survey by the Centers for Disease Control and Prevention found

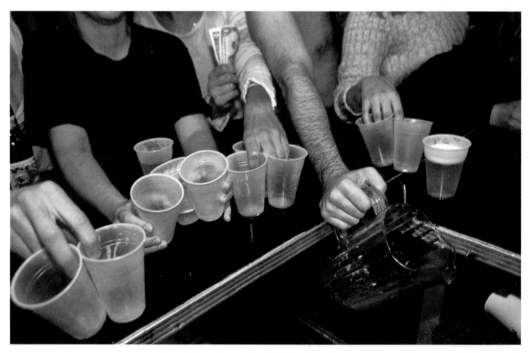

Statistics show alcohol is the drug most used by America's youth.

that 42 percent of high school students had drank some form of alcohol in the previous month, 28 percent had ridden in a car with someone who had been drinking, and 10 percent had gotten behind the wheel after drinking.

What Is Alcohol?

So, what exactly is this substance that can cause so much harm to those who use it? There are many different nicknames for—and different types of—alcohol, so it is easy to become confused when one is mentioned. Brew, cold ones, and suds? Booze, hard stuff, and hooch? Juice, sauce, and liquor? All of these are slang terms for alcohol.

However, there are only three main classifications of alcohol. Each classification has many subcategories and varieties, and the alcohol content of each one varies greatly. In general, those three classifications are

BEERS, which are most commonly made from four basic ingredients: malted grains, hops, yeast, and water

WINES, which are made from different types of fruits (most frequently grapes) and yeast

SPIRITS, also known as "hard liquor" or "hard

alcohol," which are made from grains and fruits, as well as some vegetables, and yeast

The alcohol in beer, wine, and spirits is created through a process called **fermentation**. In this process, grains, fruits, or vegetables are introduced to bacteria or yeast, which turn those foods' sugars into alcohol.

With all the negatives and uncertainties associated with drinking, the most obvious question is, "Why do teens drink alcohol?" Turns out, there

Alcohol is broken down into three main categories: beers, wines, and spirits.

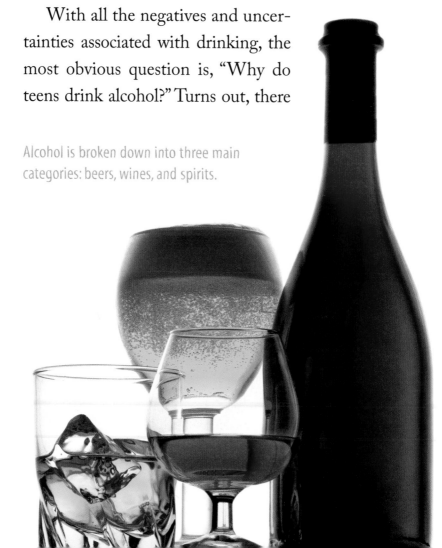

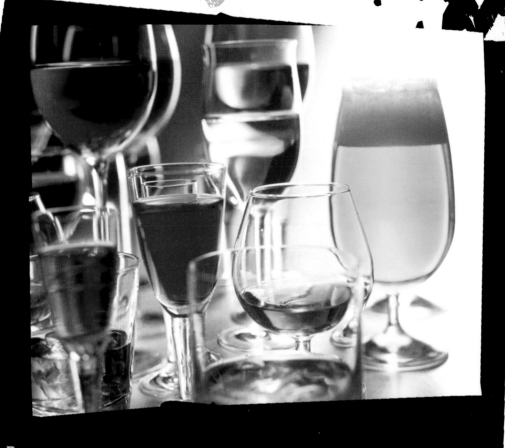

WHAT IS ONE DRINK?

Because alcohol content differs from drink to drink, exactly what makes up one serving of alcohol differs, depending on the type of drink. Beer typically is between 4 and 8 percent alcohol, and the average serving size is 12 ounces. Wine usually is about 10 to 22 percent alcohol, and one serving is 5 ounces. Hard alcohol is usually about 40 to 55 percent alcohol, and a serving size—also known as a shot—is 1.5 ounces. Therefore, one 12-ounce glass of beer equals one 5-ounce glass of wine, which equals one shot of hard alcohol.

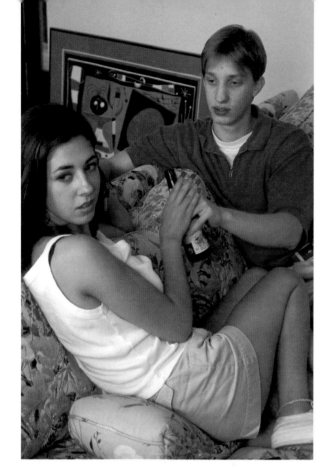
Peer pressure is one of the main reasons teens decide to drink alcohol.

are several reasons. Some do it because of **peer pressure**, out of curiosity, or to feel older. Others do it because they have bought in to television advertisements they have seen that glamorize drinking.

Some teens drink because they believe it makes them feel good or helps them relax. Koren Zailckas—a former teenage alcoholic who went on to write the best-selling book *Smashed* about her experiences—did it for another reason: "Most every girl I've known drank as an expression of her *unhappiness*," she wrote. "I too drank in no small part because I felt shamed, self-conscious, and small."

Drinking frequently as a teenager did not work out well for Zailckas. What began as a chug of alcohol with a friend during eighth grade devolved into an addiction that led to years of **binge drinking**, blackouts, brushes

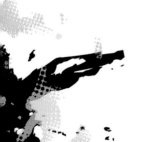

with date rape, and emergency room visits, including the time she blacked out from drinking at age sixteen:

> **I WON'T** remember the chair that wheels me down the hospital's hall, or the white cot I am lain on, or the tube that coasts through my esophagus like a snake into a crawl space. Yet I will retain those lost hours, just as my forearms will hold the singes of stranger's cigarettes in coming years, as my back will hold the scratch of a spear-point fence, as my fingers will hold griddle scars from a nonstick grill. This is the first of many forgotten injuries that will imprint me just the same.

Zailckas eventually quit drinking. Millions of other Americans who start drinking—and many teens who have been through experiences as bad as or worse than Zaikcas's—will never stop. Sometimes, they will not be seriously harmed by their decision to drink. Sometimes they—and often others—will.

CHAPTER TWO

All about Alcohol

ALCOHOL CAN HAVE SEVERAL NEGATIVE effects on a developing teen's body. This makes drinking it, even in small doses, dangerous. To understand why that is the case, it is important to understand alcohol's effects on the human body.

Alcohol is a **depressant**; that is, it works on the body in the same way a tranquilizer—a medicine given to relax people—does. From the moment a person drinks alcohol, the body begins to break it down. It passes from the stomach to the small intestine, and then is absorbed into the bloodstream. As it travels throughout the body in the blood, alcohol affects everything it comes in contact with, especially the brain.

Alcohol's toll

Drinking too much alcohol over a long period of time can adversely affect nearly every part of your body. Some of the effects on major organs:

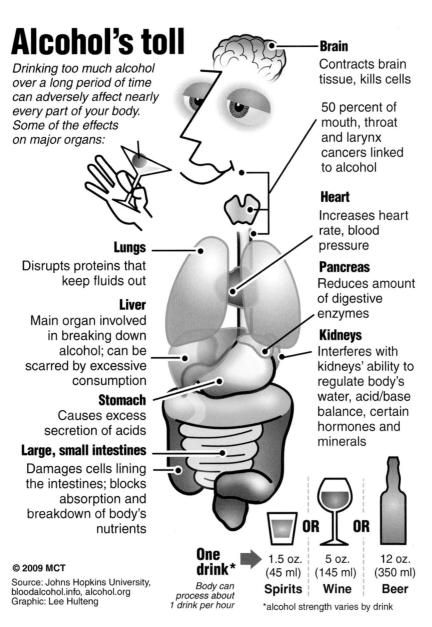

Brain
Contracts brain tissue, kills cells

50 percent of mouth, throat and larynx cancers linked to alcohol

Heart
Increases heart rate, blood pressure

Pancreas
Reduces amount of digestive enzymes

Kidneys
Interferes with kidneys' ability to regulate body's water, acid/base balance, certain hormones and minerals

Lungs
Disrupts proteins that keep fluids out

Liver
Main organ involved in breaking down alcohol; can be scarred by excessive consumption

Stomach
Causes excess secretion of acids

Large, small intestines
Damages cells lining the intestines; blocks absorption and breakdown of body's nutrients

© 2009 MCT
Source: Johns Hopkins University, bloodalcohol.info, alcohol.org
Graphic: Lee Hulteng

One drink*
Body can process about 1 drink per hour

Spirits	Wine	Beer
1.5 oz. (45 ml)	5 oz. (145 ml)	12 oz. (350 ml)

OR   OR

*alcohol strength varies by drink

This diagram illustrates alcohol's effects on the human body.

Once alcohol is in the bloodstream, it can be measured. This measurement is called the **blood alcohol concentration** (BAC). Initially, those who drink alcohol will feel what is known as a "buzz," or a mild **euphoria**. Although alcohol is indeed a depressant, during the buzz stage of drinking, it often makes people behave as if they have taken the opposite of a typical depressant. They become more talkative, outgoing, and relaxed. Some people become more confident and less anxious. This is one of the main reasons adults over the legal drinking age of twenty-one choose to consume alcohol.

As more alcohol is consumed, BAC rises, and a depressant effect replaces the euphoria. Drinkers soon become sleepy and have trouble understanding or remembering things. Their reaction time slows, their vision blurs, and they begin to lose their balance. With more drinking, things get worse. Confusion sets in, and speech becomes slurred. Add even more alcohol, and people become unconscious, their body temperature decreases, and their breathing becomes shallower. Those with BACs of more than 0.5 percent (one-half of 1 percent) usually stop breathing and die. But reactions to alcohol can vary, depending on the individual. For example, in some people, death can occur at much lower BACs.

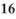

How Much Does It Take?

A person's BAC depends on several variables, including weight, number of drinks consumed, gender, the amount of food eaten, and the amount of time it took to consume the drinks. An average boy who weighs 140 pounds and had three drinks in one hour would be legally drunk, with a 0.08 BAC. An average girl who weighs 140 pounds would need to have a little more than two drinks in one hour to reach the 0.08 level.

Even if a teen were to stop drinking before any of the more severe negative effects were felt, the alcohol might still have caused long-term harm. The teen brain is far different than the adult brain because it still is developing. According to *Just Say Know*, a book about alcohol written by three doctors, introducing alcohol into the body during the teen years could change the brain's wiring "in unpredictable ways for the rest of a person's life." The doctors' research showed that "teens shouldn't drink because their brains are more sensitive.... [They are] more vulnerable to the effects of alcohol on mental function."

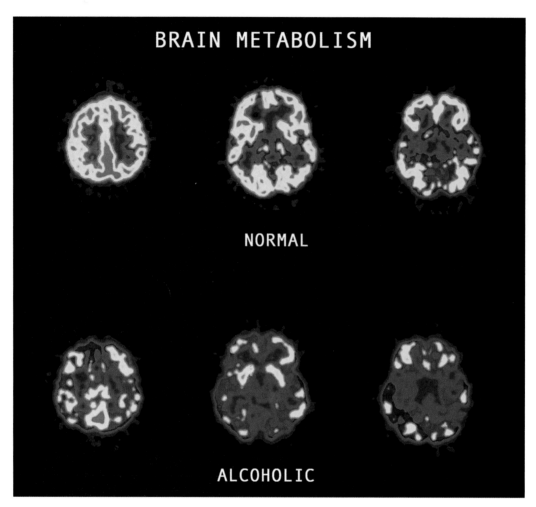

BRAIN METABOLISM

NORMAL

ALCOHOLIC

A scan compares brain function in a non-drinker (top) and an alcoholic (bottom). The lack of the yellow indicator color shows abnormal brain function in the alcoholic.

Some studies suggest that drinking as a teenager can cause irreversible brain damage. Teen brains also become addicted more easily than adult brains do.

18

Common Myths

Many people believe there are ways to get sober quickly, by speeding up the removal of alcohol from the system. None of them work. In truth, only time can remove alcohol from the body. It can take two or three hours for the alcohol in one drink to leave a person's system. Still, many people believe they can clear the alcohol from their systems faster using certain tricks. Some common methods people believe can make them sober faster include

- drinking coffee, soda, or another form of caffeine
- sleeping
- exercising
- taking a cold shower
- drinking water

The Many Cons

Potentially causing harm to a developing teen brain is not the only negative effect of drinking alcohol. Youth who drink alcohol also are more likely to experience

- school problems, such as lower grades and more absences
- social problems, such as getting into fights

- unplanned sexual activity, leading to unwanted pregnancies
- higher homicide and suicide risks
- alcohol-related car crashes
- injuries such as burns and falls
- drowning

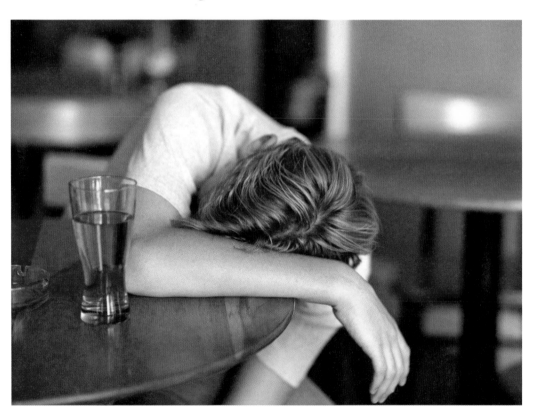

Alcohol consumption comes with a heavy price, such as negative effects on the brain, social problems, and injuries.

In addition to the brain, many of the body's other organs are affected by drinking alcohol. Drinking can lead to irregular heartbeats, high blood pressure, and heart failure. Large amounts of alcohol can also damage the liver and stomach, weaken the immune system, and might lead to certain types of cancer.

Binge Drinking

About 90 percent of the alcohol consumed by people under the age of twenty-one is during episodes of binge drinking. Binge drinking is commonly associated with college students, but is done by people of all ages. Drinking large amounts of alcohol in one sitting automatically raises a person's BAC beyond the buzz level and into the harmful zone. One study found that 63 percent of college students who binge drank had done something they later regretted. Fifty-four percent said they had forgotten where they went or what they did. Forty-two percent said they had unplanned sexual activity during their binge, and 21 percent said they had unprotected sex, which itself presents many health risks.

A 2010 study by the U.S. Department of Agriculture said there are no health benefits to binge drinking.

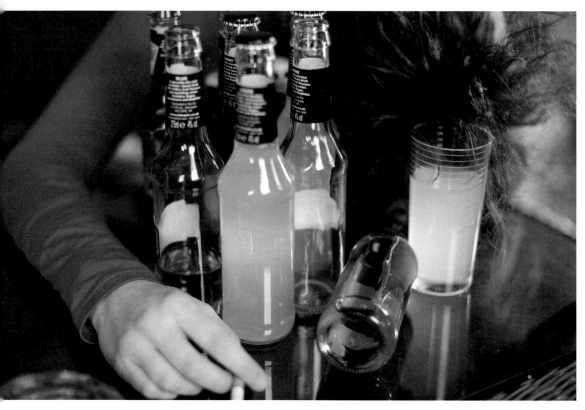

Drinking multiple alcoholic beverages in one sitting is termed "binge drinking."

The study also said binge drinking "increases the risk of cirrhosis of the liver, hypertension, stroke, type 2 diabetes, cancer of the upper gastrointestinal tract and colon, injury, and violence. . . . Excessive alcohol consumption is responsible for an average of 79,000 deaths in the United States each year. More than half of these deaths are due to binge drinking."

WEIGHT GAIN

Another negative side effect of drinking alcohol that concerns many teens is weight gain. Alcohol is a liquid, but that does not mean it is calorie-free. And, because it is easier to consume than, say, a slice of pizza, people often end up forgetting about the calories it contains. This leads to them taking in more calories from alcohol—often mixed with other drinks, such as soda and sugary fruit juices—than they would from solid food. Worst of all, alcohol has little nutritional value, so it does not provide the micronutrients the drinker needs to stay healthy.

Alcohol poisoning, which results in near-immediate death, is another by-product of binge drinking. It is what happened to Julia Gonzalez, a sixteen-year-old from California who was found dead in a park in late December 2007. The cause of her death initially was a mystery, because her body showed no signs of physical injury or assault. A toxicology report revealed that Gonzalez's BAC was 0.52, six and a half times higher than the legal limit for intoxication.

The coroner who issued the report said that, at only 5 feet 2 inches tall and about 100 pounds, Gonzalez would have needed to consume about sixteen alcoholic drinks in one hour for that much to be in her system when she died. Doctor Richard Clark, director of toxicology at the University of California at San Diego, said Gonzalez probably slipped into a coma. Then she either stopped breathing or her heart stopped pumping—or both. He said, "As with all sedatives, and alcohol is a heavy sedative, the body slowly shuts down."

Alcohol depresses nerves that control breathing and the gag reflex. Because alcohol irritates the stomach, it also is common for those who drink it to vomit. The combination of vomiting and a depressed gag reflex means that it is easy for those who vomit while drunk to choke and die. Many stars have died that way, including legendary musicians and actors.

Gateway Drug?

The indirect impacts of alcohol sometimes can be just as dangerous as the direct ones. Many experts believe alcohol is a gateway drug; that is, it often is the first step toward the use of other, harder drugs, such as cocaine and heroin. Others disagree with the gateway assessment, saying too many factors contribute to teens' uses of hard drugs to blame

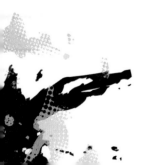

SIGNS OF ALCOHOL POISONING

Being able to recognize the signs of alcohol poisoning is critical for getting a sick person treatment before it is too late. Signs of acute alcohol poisoning include

- vomiting
- seizures
- slow or irregular breathing
- mental confusion, stupor, or coma
- pale or bluish skin color
- low body temperature
- unconsciousness

it on just alcohol use. Regardless, combining alcohol with any other drugs—including some over-the-counter cold medicines or even caffeine—is extremely dangerous and can even be fatal.

In 2010 an alcoholic beverage called Four Loko found its way into the national spotlight for combining two drugs in one drink. The fruit-flavored drink, marketed in bright-colored 23.5-ounce cans, contained as much alcohol as

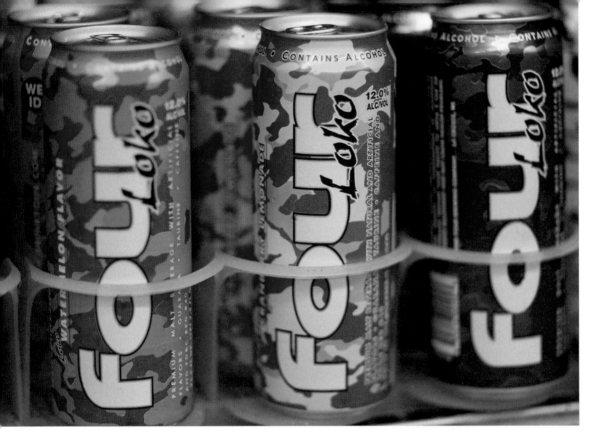

The U.S. Food and Drug Administration banned Four Loko, a caffeinated and alcoholic drink, and others like it.

four beers and as much caffeine as three cups of coffee. The combination of depressant and stimulant made it difficult for those who drank it to tell how much alcohol they really had drank. The drink gained the dubious nickname "blackout in a can."

Cyndra Krogen-Morton, a health educator at Sacramento State University in California, said, "The caffeine keeps them awake and wanting to drink more, when alcohol without the caffeine would have just made

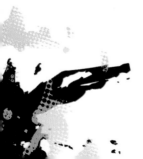

The makers of Four Loko were not the first alcohol company to use marketing tricks to entice younger people to drink their product. Such tactics have been used for decades. But the media frenzy that resulted from Four Loko's troubles even got high-ranking

GOVERNMENT STEPS IN

politicians involved in the matter. Senator Charles Schumer of New York, for example, wrote a letter to the Federal Trade Commission asking it to crack down on companies that seemed to be marketing alcoholic beverages to teens. He said the brightly colored cans of drinks such as Four Loko are designed to attract young people. He wrote, "Any practices that target alcohol advertising to underage drinkers must be stopped."

Four Loko and similar caffeinated alcoholic drinks were subsequently banned by the U.S. Food and Drug Administration. The makers of Four Loko soon removed all caffeine from their beverage but continued selling the product.

them tired. The stimulation mixed with alcohol really sets people up for alcohol poisoning." Soon, Four Loko was being blamed for hospitalizations and deaths across the United States. One high-profile case involved a twenty-year-old Florida college student named Jason Keiran. According to his family, Keiran drank at least three cans of Four Loko before accidentally shooting himself in the head. Kieran's accident was fatal, and his family sued the makers of Four Loko.

Learning about the way alcohol works and its impact on the body makes one wonder even more why anyone would want to drink it. Most people would admit that drinking a depressing, weight-swelling, potentially poisonous and fatal substance does not sound like a smart thing to do. Yet even people teens look up to—including their parents and famous celebrities—continue to drink.

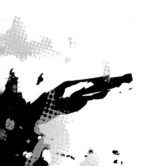

CHAPTER THREE

Real Stories

CELEBRITIES APPEAR TO HAVE IT ALL. On TV, they star in hit shows. In movies, they play funny, strong, or tough characters. In magazines, they pose for pretty portraits, wearing the latest designer fashions. Sometimes it is easy to forget there are real people behind the images. But those stars have flaws, just as regular people do. Sometimes, those flaws involve using too much alcohol. Actress Lindsay Lohan was one such star.

Lohan starred in her first major movie at age eleven, playing the roles of the twin sisters in *The Parent Trap*. Before her twentieth birthday, the freckled redhead was a household name, having starred in several other films, including *Freaky Friday*, *Mean Girls*, *Herbie Fully Loaded*, and

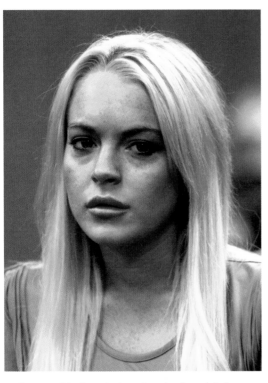

Actress Lindsay Lohan has had multiple run-ins with the law due to her abuse of alcohol.

A Prairie Home Companion. Her performances had made her millions of dollars. It appeared as if nothing could dim Lohan's rising star—except for her self-destructive behavior.

At some point during her rise to fame, Lohan began smoking cigarettes and drinking alcohol. When she was seventeen, she began attending Alcoholics Anonymous (A.A.) meetings. When that news became public in 2006, the then eighteen-year-old Lohan told *People* magazine, "I drink with my friends at home, but there's no need to. I feel better not drinking. It's more fun." Despite her words, Lohan did not stop drinking, and many problems—personal and legal—have followed.

Lohan is not the only young star whose life has been negatively impacted by alcohol. Actor Drew Barrymore's career also was derailed by alcohol at a young age. Before she was fourteen years old, the star of *E.T.: The Extra-*

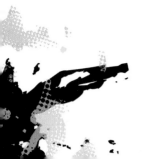

Terrestrial had smoked cigarettes, used alcohol and other drugs, and completed a trip to **rehabilitation**. In her 1990 book, *Little Girl Lost*, Barrymore wrote:

> **I STARTED** drinking with friends when I slept over at their houses. Just sneaking a drink here, a beer there. After a while, though, drinking became the only way I thought I could have fun. Only I didn't drink to have fun. I drank to get drunk.

Later, Barrymore progressed to smoking marijuana and inhaling cocaine, saying that alcohol had become boring to her. For her, alcohol was a gateway drug. Barrymore eventually overcame her addictions to star in several blockbuster films as an adult.

Recently, popular young celebrities such as Miley Cyrus and Britney Spears have been linked to excessive alcohol use. Cyrus, who will not turn twenty-one until November 2013, has been photographed drinking alcohol numerous times. Spears has long battled issues with drugs and alcohol. In 2008 her mother, Lynne Spears, wrote a book, *Through the Storm*, about her famous daughters,

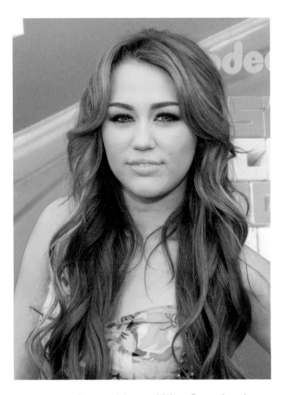

Actress/singer Miley Cyrus has been photographed drinking alcohol when she was underage.

Britney and her actor sister, Jamie Lynn. In the book, Lynne Spears wrote that Britney first started drinking at age thirteen and progressed to harder drugs shortly thereafter. Since that time, Britney has had several run-ins with the law and has been to rehab a few times.

Celebrity DUIs

On occasion, alcohol use has gotten celebrities into serious trouble. Actor Tracy Morgan of *Saturday Night Live* and *30 Rock* fame has been arrested for driving under the influence of alcohol (DUI) more than once. After his second arrest, he said, "Driving under the influence isn't cool. I have kids and I don't want anyone to get the wrong message about that. It's something I've resolved in my life. Things got a little bumpy and it was taken care of." Khloe Kardashian, Shia LaBeouf, Paris Hilton, Trace Adkins, and many other

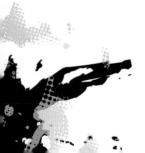

celebs also have been cited for DUIs. In many instances, the negative publicity the stars have received for doing so has damaged or even ended their careers.

The fact that celebrities are arrested for DUIs should not be surprising; there are more than one million DUI arrests in the United States each year. In 2008 there were 37,261 alcohol-related traffic fatalities, which means at least one person directly involved in the accident (driver

Staying Safe

Although it seems obvious that you should never get into a car driven by someone who has been drinking, saying no to such a ride is not always easy. Partnership for a Drug-Free America suggests responding with one of the following excuses:

- "No thanks. I already called my mom for a ride. She said she'd give you one, too. You should take her up on it. We can come back for your car tomorrow."
- "No way. You're wasted! With my luck, you'll puke on me in the car. I'll hitch a ride with someone else, thanks."
- "You look pretty drunk to me! And any cop that pulls us over will think so, too. Sorry, it's not worth the risk."

or pedestrian) had some amount of alcohol in his or her system. The number of yearly alcohol-impaired traffic fatalities, meaning someone involved had a blood alcohol concentration (BAC) of 0.08 or higher, was 11,773, or more than 32 per day.

A Deadly Crash

Though the celebrity cases are the ones most people remember, most of the thirty-two daily alcohol-impaired traffic fatalities that take place across the United States do not receive much fanfare. That does not mean each one is not impactful in its own way. To those in the city of Olathe, Kansas, Benjamin Denham's accident certainly was.

In March 2010 the eighteen-year-old was driving with two teenage friends in Overland Park, Kansas, when tragedy struck. Denham was driving more than 100 miles per hour when he lost control of his Cadillac. The car hit a power pole and a garage before it rolled and burst into flames. A witness pulled Denham from the car and saved his life. But the two passengers, Olathe High School students ages eighteen and seventeen, died in the wreck.

Denham had a history of drinking and driving. On this occasion, his BAC was nearly twice the legal limit.

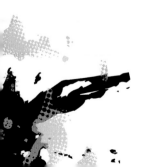

34

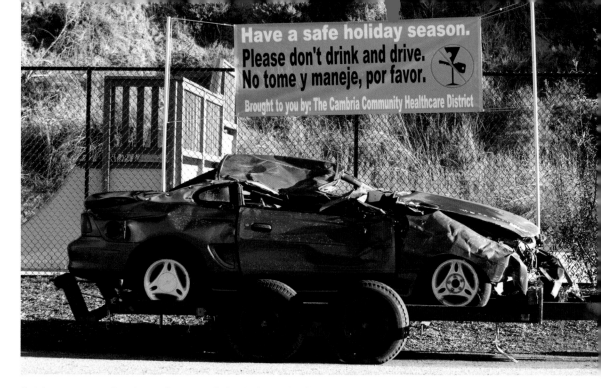

Driving a car under the influence of alcohol can lead to injury and even death. This vehicle was in an accident in which someone was drinking and driving.

The judge sentenced him to almost nine years in prison. Denham's father spoke at his son's sentencing. He said his son was guilt-ridden and had faced many surgeries due to the accident, and his body was covered in scars. The father said his son "believes his scars can be used to warn other kids." Earlier, Denham's mother had said, "It was the worst moment of our lives to tell him about his friends. It took two hours; we wept with him. He is sorry he can't redo that decision."

There are many agencies working hard to show teens that drinking can—and often does—have some very real consequences, as it did in Denham's case. Massachusetts General Hospital's Trauma Center, for example, uses a high-tech simulator that re-creates the front of a car. Teens enter the simulator and start driving, sober at first. Then the simulator gradually increases the teens' "alcohol level," making it harder to steer and brake. Sandy Muse, a nurse practitioner working with the program, said, "Teenagers think they're invincible like some adults do, as well, and we're trying to get the message through to high school kids that drunk driving is no joke."

Teens do not need to be driving to be penalized for drinking alcohol. In addition to dealing with upset parents, teens can be kicked off sports teams or out of school. They also can be cited by police for various criminal offenses, including for being a **minor in possession** (MIP). Those cited as MIPs also can lose their driver's licenses, even if they were not driving at the time, and can receive various fines. In most areas, a teen does not even have to be in possession of alcohol to get arrested for an MIP. Simply having a little bit of alcohol in the body or appearing drunk is enough to get arrested. The most important thing teens must ask before taking a sip is, "Is this worth the risk?"

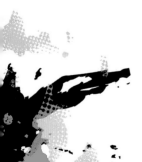

CHAPTER FOUR

Staying Sober

THE EVER-PRESENT NATURE OF ALCOHOL in American society often makes it appear as though everyone is a drinker. In 2009 about 130.6 million Americans ages twelve or older said they were current drinkers, meaning they had consumed alcohol at least once in the previous thirty days. Those numbers included 10.4 million children ages twelve to twenty that were doing so illegally. So *is* everyone doing it?

The 130.6 million people mentioned above represent a little more than half the entire population of the country. That means a little less than half of Americans are not current drinkers. The 10.4 million youth drinkers represent just 27.2 percent of people in that age group, meaning only about one out of four in that age group currently drinks. Most people in that group are able to withstand peer pressure, do not cave in to television ads, overlook their family members' drinking, and steer clear of any alcohol in their homes. There are many ways they do this.

The most basic way they avoid alcohol is by just saying "no." That is what fifteen-year-old Tabor Smith of Greenwood Village, Colorado, did in 2009 when a friend offered him a drink from a bottle of vodka during a house party. "It didn't seem like a big deal to take a drink from the bottle, but I knew it wasn't a good idea for me," he told *Scholastic Choices* magazine. "[I said] 'No thanks, I have to go home later and my parents will be there.'" Without drinking, he said he still "had just as much fun as the others did without getting sick from drinking."

When he was a high school freshman, Ricky Birt of Springfield, Ohio, did something similar. Happy to be invited to a party that many popular students were going to, Birt was told everyone there would be playing a drinking game. He turned down the invite. He told *Scholastic Choices*, "When I really thought about it, there was nothing to draw me to the party except for the wrong reasons." Some of those who attended the party, Birt said, ended up

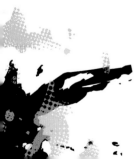

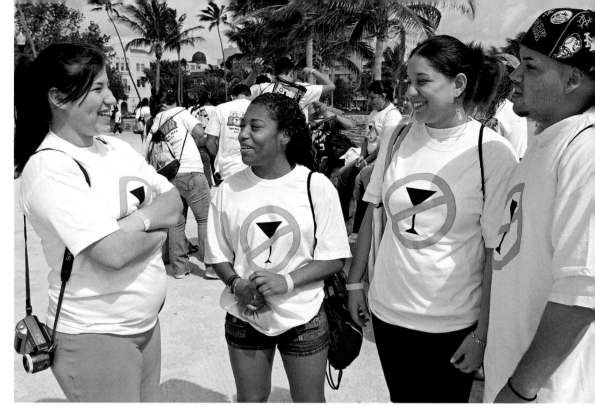

Drug Free Youth in Town volunteers promote a sober spring break in Miami, Florida.

driving drunk and were pulled over by police and arrested. Birt was happy he did not end up in that situation. "They could have killed someone or hurt themselves," he said.

How to Say No

Exactly *how* to say no to offers of alcohol—as the teens mentioned above did—is often the biggest hurdle for teens to overcome. The truth is, there are as many ways to decline alcohol as there are reasons for saying no. According to the TeensHealth website, teens just need to find out what works best for them. "Some find it helps to say no without giving an explanation; others think that offering their reasons works better," the site says. Such reasons can be as simple as "I'm not into drinking" or as specific as "I have a game tomorrow" or "My uncle died from drinking." A teen can also place the blame on his or her parents or another adult, if necessary.

Volunteering to be the designated driver is another way for teens to say no without actually having to utter the word. Another method of avoiding the drinking question is carrying around a cup filled with soda. In that case, no one will likely know or ask what the person is drinking and will assume that he or she is drinking alcohol.

One of the best ways for teens to steer clear of alcohol, reported TeensHealth, is to plan a "just say no" strategy long before the need arises. "You and a friend can develop a signal for when it's time to leave, for example. You can also make sure that you have plans to do something besides just hanging out in someone's basement drinking beer all night," the site says. Suggested alternative activities included trips to the movies, a concert, or a sporting event.

In his book *Reality Gap*, Stephen Wallace stresses the importance of practicing what to say before it comes time to say it. Wallace, chairman of the group Students Against

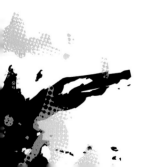

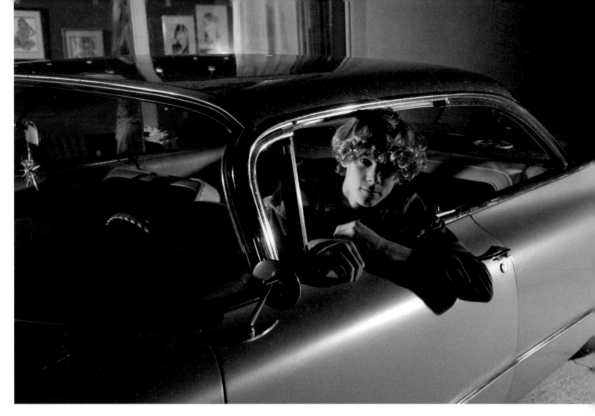

One way to say "no" to alcohol is to volunteer to be the designated driver when out with friends.

Destructive Decisions (SADD), writes, "Like a football player practicing a fumble drill or a firefighter practicing a rescue, teens who think through role-play responses to tough situations are more likely to do what they want to do than to make a split-second error in judgment due to peer pressure."

Reasons Teens Drink

With so many young people breaking the law to drink alcohol, it is logical to wonder why they do so. The reasons

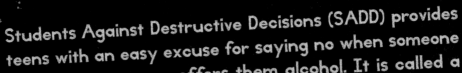

CONTRACT FOR LIFE

Students Against Destructive Decisions (SADD) provides teens with an easy excuse for saying no when someone offers them alcohol. It is called a Contract for Life. The contract is between a teen and his or her parent. Under the contract, the teen promises to stay alcohol—and drug—free, to never drive under the influence, to never ride with someone who is under the influence, to always wear a seat belt, and to always call the parent if the teen is in a bad situation. In turn, the parent also promises to not drive under the influence and always wear a seat belt, to provide safe transportation anytime his or her child should ask for it, and to wait to discuss the situation until the heat of the moment has passed.

teens drink are nearly as numerous as the types of alcohol available to them. Some of the reasons are social. Others are environmental or personal.

Peer pressure is a big factor in why teens decide to drink and also in the amount they drink when they do so. Matthew Sunshine was a nineteen-year-old college freshman at Northwestern University, in Illinois, in June 2008. He had just finished a final exam when he and a friend decided to celebrate by drinking alcohol. Within an hour, said his father, Sunshine drank seventeen shots of vodka. It would only have taken three or four to make him legally drunk. But Sunshine's father, Jeff Sunshine, said peer pressure caused his son to drink more and faster than he otherwise would have. "There were eight to ten Northwestern students who wandered in and out of the room who were sober, to come watch this [and] cheer it on," Jeff Sunshine said.

After Sunshine passed out, friends put him to bed. Some people drew pictures on his face with markers. Sometime in the next few hours, Sunshine died from alcohol poisoning.

Everyone likes to fit in and be accepted. Such acceptance helps boost self-esteem and gives people an identity. Adults are not excluded from this pressure, but finding acceptance is more important with teens than with any other age group. It is a natural part of growing up. According to the therapist and author Stephen G. Biddulph, it often is easiest for teens looking for acceptance to find it among groups who drink and use drugs because those groups "are often less discriminating and selective. The only requirement to entrance into the group

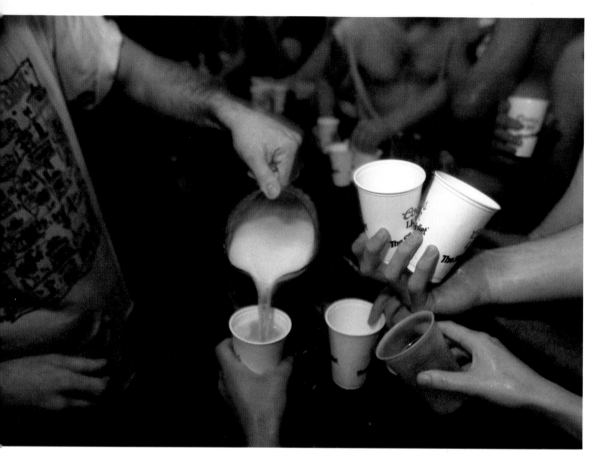

Some teens choose to fit in by choosing groups of friends that drink.

is to use and perhaps participate in the activities associated with the drug use." Anyone can qualify.

Peer pressure is often subtle. It is not always obvious that teens are being pressured. Sometimes, drinking "just happens." Also, peer pressure can work in a positive way.

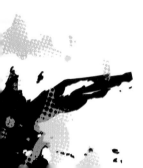

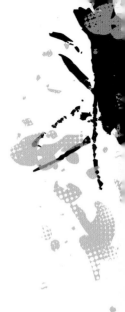

Those who do not use alcohol can have as great an influence on a teen's actions as those who do drink.

Some teens begin drinking because their parents or other family members do. Children who live in homes where the parents drink alcohol are more likely to view drinking as an acceptable behavior. They see it at the dinner table. They see Dad sitting in front of the television with a beer or Mom sitting on the patio with a glass of wine, book in hand. In the majority of cases, teens are first introduced to alcohol either through a family member or by someone else in their home. If alcohol in the home is in a place where kids can easily access it, they are more likely to try it. The 2010 National Survey on Drug Abuse and Health showed that almost half of kids ages twelve to fourteen who drink get their alcohol for free from a family member or at home.

Certain medical conditions, such as depression and bipolar disorder, can make a teen more susceptible to first trying, and then becoming hooked on, alcohol or other drugs. They see alcohol as a way to self-medicate. Some people also are genetically predisposed to becoming addicted to such substances. In those cases, it is even more important for teens to avoid trying alcohol in the first place.

Many people believe the media also plays a big role in teen drinking. In 2009 the average person ages twelve to twenty saw an alcohol advertisement on television one time per day. That was a 71 percent increase over 2001. Exposure to such ads increases the likelihood that those who see them will start drinking or will drink more if they already are drinking.

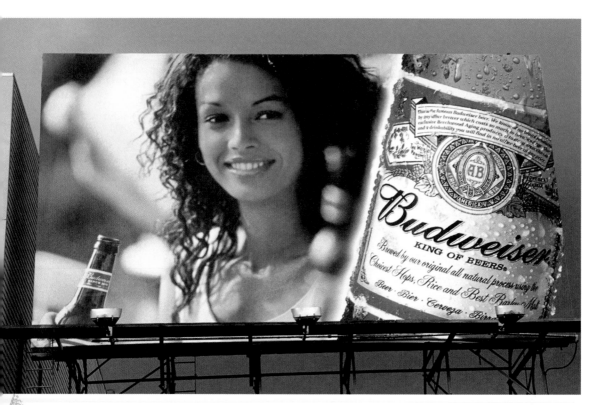

Some people believe media influence is a big reason why teens choose to drink alcohol.

Teens drink for several other reasons, as well. Those reasons include boredom, curiosity, rebellion, thrill seeking, being left unsupervised too often, and many more. Frequently, there is more than one reason. Researchers have come to realize that certain teens—such as those doing poorly in school and those with peers who drink—are more likely to drink than others. Likewise, there are those who are less likely to drink, especially those whose friends do not drink and whose parents monitor them closely.

Alcoholism

Despite their best attempts at abstaining, teens often do get involved with alcohol. Those who drink too much risk becoming addicted. **Alcoholism**, also known as alcohol dependence, can affect people of any age. Common signs of alcoholism include

- not being able to control how often or how much alcohol is consumed
- tolerance, meaning it takes more and more alcohol to feel the same effect
- **withdrawal** symptoms, such as sickness, sweating, shakiness, and anxiety when

alcohol is withheld

- quitting once-enjoyable activities in order to drink
- drinking in the morning or alone
- feeling guilty after drinking

Some people are able to overcome alcoholism on their own. Others need help. There are many options for those who are addicted to alcohol. Help is easy to find. Alcoholics Anonymous (A.A.) is one organization. A.A. has been offering help to problem drinkers since 1935 and has chapters in more than 180 countries. The basis of A.A. is its twelve-step program. The first step is to admit that alcohol has control of one's life. Other steps include making a list of everyone the person with the drinking problem has harmed and working to make amends with each of them. As its name indicates, A.A. is confidential. Members who attend meetings often use only their first names. Some choose not to speak but rather to observe and listen. The program is not affiliated with any religion, is free, and is open to people of all ages.

Kevin was one teen who benefited from the program, which he joined when he was fourteen. "I have had two overwhelming spiritual experiences in my life," Kevin said

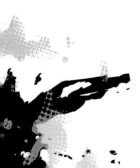

in an A.A. brochure called "Young People and A.A." "The second was when I decided to get sober. The first was when I took my first drink. . . . That was the best drink I ever had—and I would spend my drinking career trying to recreate it." Kevin was unable to do so. His drinking caused him to become a habitual liar. He overdosed on alcohol and ran away from home. Finally, he joined A.A. In 2007, the year the pamphlet was published, Kevin celebrated his nineteenth year of sobriety. "I have not found it necessary to tempt fate again," he said.

Rehab

For those who are not able to kick a drinking habit on their own or with the help of an organization such as A.A., rehabilitation, or rehab, programs are another option. Rehab is a term that often is thrown around in conversations, but it can have a few meanings. Some rehab centers are inpatient facilities, meaning the patients live on the premises. Others are outpatient facilities, where people go to receive treatment on a regular basis but continue to live at home. Some programs focus on religion, while others are secular. Some patients are there voluntarily; others are ordered to go there by the court system.

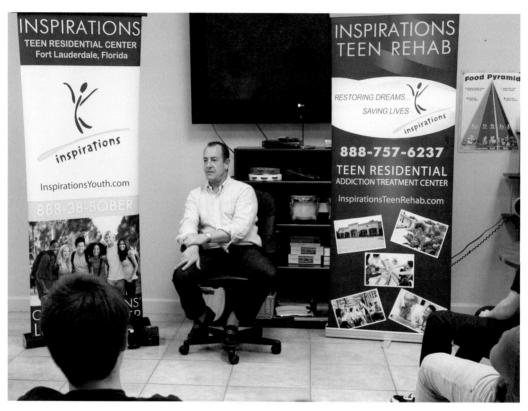

Lindsay Lohan's father, Michael, speaks to teens at Inspirations Teen Rehab in Fort Lauderdale, Florida, about the dangers of teenage substance abuse.

In almost all circumstances, rehab programs use counselors to help those who are dependent on alcohol or other drugs overcome their addictions. Rehab is not easy. At the Visions Adolescent Treatment Center in Malibu, California, patients are subjected to random drug testing throughout their stay, made to attend school for

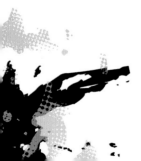

three hours each day, five days a week, and have to take part in counseling groups that teach strategies for stress management, anger management, and more. The teens are directed by teams of therapists, nurses, medical doctors, psychiatrists, and others. The facility is located in a rural setting on 12 acres of wooded land, and the gate to the area is locked. The minimum amount of time those admitted to the program must stay is forty-five days.

Although it works a lot of the time, rehab is definitely not a cure-all. Not all teens successfully complete such programs. Others may complete programs, but have difficulty once they are back "on the outside" and have to deal with situations where alcohol is involved on their own.

There are programs for teens who are not addicted to alcohol but are deeply affected by people who are. **Alateen** is such a program. Alateen is a branch of **Al-Anon**, an organization designed to help families and friends of alcoholics cope with the problems that stem from dealing with or living with an alcoholic. Alateen is specifically for teens dealing with such issues, while Al-Anon is geared toward everyone in an affected family. Both groups hold regular meetings and adhere to principles similar to those of A.A. Those who attend Alateen meetings have said they do so mostly because their mental health and well-being are greatly affected by those they know who drink. In 2006 the average age of an Alateen member in the United States was fourteen, and 65 percent of members were female. Nearly three out of four members had joined Alateen because either a parent's or stepparent's drinking had influenced them to do so. One out of seven Alateen members said they also were members of Alcoholics Anonymous.

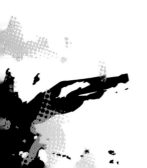

CHAPTER FIVE

Knowledge Is Key

THE NUMBERS ARE STRAIGHTFORWARD.
Most teens choose to try alcohol before they graduate high school. Yet, after trying it, most teens choose not to drink alcohol regularly. If it is as great as it is often said to be, why not?

According to those millions of teens who choose to not drink, there are many reasons. One study conducted by the University of New Hampshire asked kids to name the main reason they did not drink alcohol. These are the results.

"I don't want to mess up my body."
—34 percent

"I don't need it to make me happy."
—20 percent

"My school, athletic, or work
performance would suffer."
—16 percent

"I might become an alcoholic."
—8 percent

"I'm afraid of what I would do or
say under the influence."
—6 percent

The remainder of those polled either said it was because their parents did not approve, they believe drinking is morally wrong, or that their friends did not approve.

Across the country, there is even a subculture of young people who have made lifelong promises not to drink, smoke cigarettes, or use illegal drugs. People who do so are

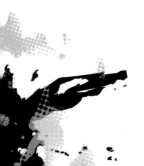

called straight edge. The movement was named after a song written in 1980 by the punk rock band Minor Threat. Today, straight edgers often draw or tattoo Xs on their hands to let people know who they are.

Teens armed with the facts about the dangers of drinking alcohol—that it is a poisonous, dangerous, illegal, and potentially deadly substance—are less likely to do it. They do not want to increase their risk of committing suicide, drowning, gaining weight, or dying in a car accident. They do not want an unwanted pregnancy, a criminal record, or to spend several weeks

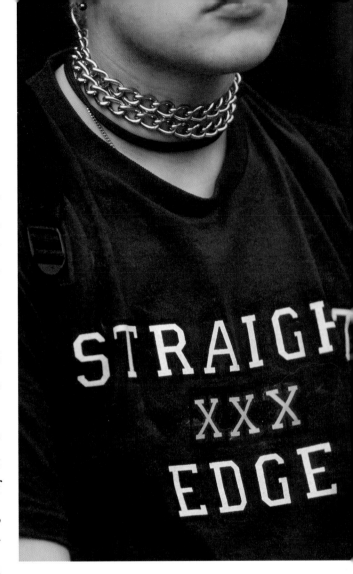

A straight edge member shows off the movement's logo and symbols.

in a rehab facility. They know about addiction and that drinking alcohol could very well lead them to that point.

Teens who do not drink alcohol listen to the advice given by experts who know what alcohol is all about.

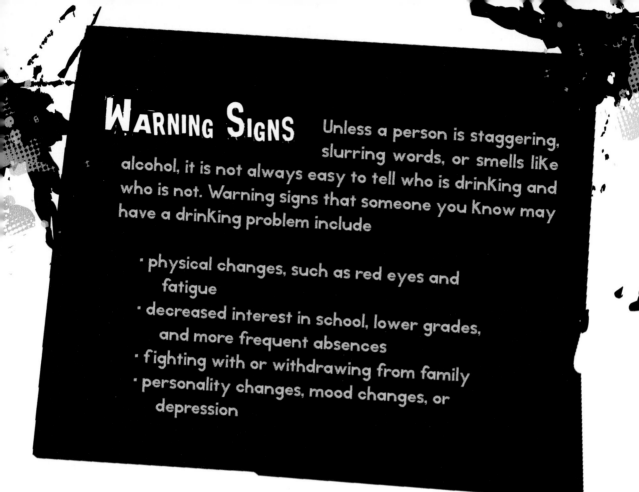

WARNING SIGNS

Unless a person is staggering, slurring words, or smells like alcohol, it is not always easy to tell who is drinking and who is not. Warning signs that someone you know may have a drinking problem include

- physical changes, such as red eyes and fatigue
- decreased interest in school, lower grades, and more frequent absences
- fighting with or withdrawing from family
- personality changes, mood changes, or depression

They read and believe websites such as KidsHealth.org, which says, "It can be tempting to try alcohol. It's normal to be curious about new things, especially if it seems like everyone is doing it. But everyone is not drinking alcohol. Don't believe it if someone says you're immature for not drinking alcohol. You're actually more mature . . . because you're being strong and smart." Teens who do not drink alcohol listen to other teens.

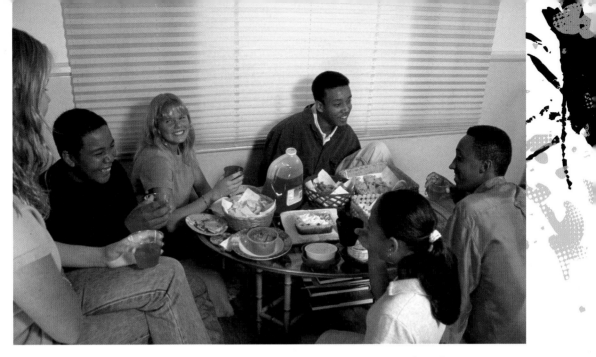
Alcohol does not need to be factored in when having a great time with friends.

"All too often it seems teenagers turn to alcohol as a crutch; they feel that it is essential to having fun and to fitting in. At a lot of high school parties, the only focal point is drinking," said Chris Perry, a senior at Saint Francis High School in Mountain View, California. "But I have been to parties where my peers are getting wasted and I can still have a great time without feeling left out. I am an outgoing individual who can have fun and be crazy without getting drunk, and my friends respect that."

Glossary

Al-Anon a support group for those affected by a person with a drinking problem

Alateen the branch of Al-Anon aimed at teens

alcoholism a disease characterized by an addictive dependency on alcohol

alcohol poisoning the condition in which a toxic amount of alcohol is consumed in a short period of time

binge drinking consuming large quantities of alcohol on a single occasion, usually defined as five or more drinks for a male and four or more drinks for a female

blood alcohol concentration the amount of alcohol in a person's blood; also known as BAC

depressant a drug that reduces nervous system activity

euphoria joy or excitement

fermentation the process that turns the sugars in fruits, vegetables, and grains into alcohol

minor in possession a criminal charge made against a person under the legal drinking age who has been caught with alcohol or has consumed it; also known as MIP

peer pressure coercion or persuasion from a person of the same age, social standing, or background as another

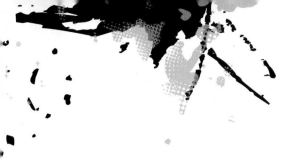

sober the state of not being drunk

rehabilitation treatment undergone by an alcoholic to
return him or her to a healthy status; also known
as rehab

withdrawal the uncomfortable mental and physical
state that occurs when a person addicted to alcohol or
another substance is kept from using it

Find Out More

Books

Aretha, David. *On the Rocks: Teens and Alcohol.* New York: Franklin Watts, 2007.

Marshall Cavendish Reference. *Drugs of Abuse.* New York: Marshall Cavendish, 2012.

Marshall Cavendish Reference. *Substance Abuse, Addiction, and Treatment.* New York: Marshall Cavendish, 2012.

Radev, Anna and KidsPeace. *I've Got This Friend Who: Advice for Teens and Their Friends on Alcohol, Drugs, Eating Disorders and More.* Center City, Minnesota: Hazelden Publishing, 2007.

DVDs

Real Life Teens: Alcohol. TMW Media Group, 2011.

Websites

Al-Anon/Alateen

www.al-anon.org

Provides information and helpful links for those of any age who are dealing with an alcoholic relative or friend.

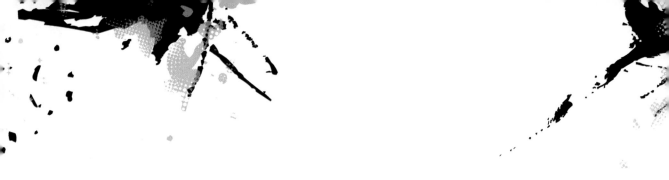

SADD (Students Against Destructive Decisions)

www.sadd.org

Offers students information on events, local gatherings, and resources that help teens help other teens make positive life decisions.

Teens Health

http://teenshealth.org/teen/

Contains links and information on a variety of teen-related topics, including a detailed section on alcohol.

The Cool Spot

www.thecoolspot.gov

Backed by various government agencies, this site offers advice on nearly every topic associated with teen drinking, including peer pressure.

Index

Pages in **boldface** are illustrations.

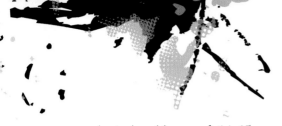

About the Author

JEFF BURLINGAME is the author of several books, including *Crystal Meth* in the Dangerous Drugs series. His books have been honored by the New York Public Library, and he has been nominated for several other awards, including a prestigious 2011 NAACP Image Award. Burlingame has won more than a dozen awards from the Society of Professional Journalists, has been a featured author on A&E's *Biography* TV series, and has lectured at various writing workshops and libraries across the Pacific Northwest.